WHAT ARE CLINICAL TRIALS?

Dr. Chardae Rodgers-Gamble

Dr. Chardae Rodgers-Gamble

Copyright © 2024 Dr. Chardae Rodgers-Gamble.

All rights reserved. No part of this book may be reproduced or transmitted in any form or by any means, electronic or mechanical, including photocopying, recording, or by any information storage and retrieval system, without written permission from the publisher.

What Are Clinical Trials?

Table of Contents

Introduction to Clinical Trials 3
Purpose of Clinical Trials 5
Phases of Clinical Trials 7
Key Players in Clinical Trials 8
Clinical Trial Design 10
Informed Consent Process 12
Recruitment and Enrollment 14
Conducting Clinical Trials 16
Data Analysis and Interpretation 18
Ethical and Regulatory Considerations 20
Benefits and Risks of Participation 22
Conclusion 24
About the Author 26

Introduction to Clinical Trials

Overview of Clinical Trials

Clinical trials are vital research studies conducted to evaluate the effectiveness and safety of new medical treatments, interventions, or devices. These trials play a crucial role in advancing medical knowledge and enhancing patient care. In essence, they provide a scientific foundation for the development and approval of new drugs and therapies by regulatory authorities such as the Food and Drug Administration (FDA). It is important to comprehend the fundamental concepts and distinctions within clinical trials, particularly the contrast between interventional and observational studies. An interventional study involves active participation by the researchers who administer a specific intervention or treatment to the participants, while an observational study entails observing and analyzing outcomes without any interference with the participants' routine. Both types contribute to the accumulation of evidence and data to drive medical progress and improve healthcare outcomes.

Historical Background

Clinical trials have a rich history dating back to ancient civilizations where various forms of experimentation were conducted to understand the effects of different treatments. The origins of clinical trials can be traced to the early efforts of physicians and scientists such as James Lind, who conducted one of the first recorded controlled clinical trials in 1747 to investigate scurvy treatments among sailors. Over time, the ethical and scientific foundations of clinical trials have evolved, leading to the development of comprehensive methodologies and regulatory frameworks.

What Are Clinical Trials?

One pivotal event in the history of clinical trials was the introduction of the Nuremberg Code in 1947, which established fundamental principles for human experimentation following the atrocities of World War II. This landmark document laid the groundwork for the ethical conduct of clinical trials and emphasized the importance of informed consent and respect for individuals participating in clinical trials. The subsequent establishment of regulatory bodies and guidelines, including the Declaration of Helsinki and the Belmont Report, further contributed to shaping the historical landscape of clinical research by prioritizing the protection of participants and the integrity of scientific investigation. Throughout history, clinical trials have played an integral role in advancing medical knowledge and improving patient care. As we delve into the historical background of clinical trials, it is crucial to recognize the significant milestones and ethical considerations that have shaped the evolution of this essential scientific practice.

Importance and Goals

By testing new treatments, interventions, or strategies, clinical trials contribute to the development of evidence-based practices that can lead to better outcomes for patients. The importance of clinical trials lies in their ability to evaluate the effectiveness and safety of potential new treatments, validate existing therapies, and explore innovative approaches to managing diseases. Through rigorous scientific methods, clinical trials generate valuable data that can influence medical guidelines, drive regulatory decisions, and shape the future of healthcare. The goals of clinical trials are multifaceted, encompassing not only the assessment of treatment efficacy and safety but also the exploration of novel therapeutic avenues and the identification of factors that may influence patient response.

Moreover, by enrolling diverse participant populations, clinical trials aim to ensure that findings are applicable across different demographic groups, ultimately striving for equitable and inclusive healthcare solutions. As such, the overarching goal of clinical trials is to translate scientific discoveries into tangible benefits for patients and society at large, ultimately striving to advance the frontiers of medicine and enhance overall public health.

What Are Clinical Trials?

Purpose of Clinical Trials

Defining the Goals of Clinical Trials

One of the primary goals of conducting clinical trials is to assess the safety and efficacy of new treatments, interventions, or drugs. By systematically gathering data through well-designed protocols, researchers aim to evaluate whether the experimental intervention offers therapeutic benefits for the target population. This includes exploring potential improvements in patient outcomes such as extended survival, enhanced quality of life, or reduced symptoms associated with the targeted condition. Furthermore, clinical trials also aim to investigate the preventive aspects of certain interventions, seeking to understand their capacity to reduce the risk of developing specific diseases or conditions. For instance, vaccine trials often focus on assessing the effectiveness of immunization in preventing infectious diseases.

In addition to therapeutic and preventative objectives, clinical trials also encompass diagnostic aims. These trials aim to evaluate the accuracy and reliability of diagnostic tools, medical devices, or imaging techniques in detecting diseases or conditions. Diagnostic trials help in identifying more effective ways of diagnosing illnesses, thereby contributing to earlier detection and timely intervention. This facet of clinical research is essential in enhancing disease detection methodologies and ultimately improving patient outcomes.

Therefore, the multifaceted goals of clinical trials resonate with the fundamental mission of advancing medical science, promoting human health, and addressing unmet medical needs. It is through these rigorous and methodical endeavors that the healthcare landscape continues to evolve, offering new hope and improved treatment paradigms for patients worldwide.

Impact of Clinical Trials on Medicine

Through meticulously designed research studies, clinical trials have contributed significantly to the development of new treatments and interventions, as well as the optimization of existing therapeutic approaches. The impact of clinical trials on medicine is multifaceted, encompassing advancements in understanding disease mechanisms, drug discovery, and evidence-based practice.

One of the primary impacts of clinical trials on medicine is the generation of robust scientific evidence. By systematically evaluating the safety and effectiveness of medical interventions in diverse patient populations, clinical trials provide crucial data that guide treatment decisions and inform clinical guidelines. This evidence-based approach not only ensures that patients receive the most appropriate and effective therapies but also promotes the rational use of healthcare resources. Moreover, clinical trials often lead to the identification of novel biomarkers, molecular targets, and diagnostic tools, which can revolutionize disease detection and management.

Furthermore, the influence of clinical trials extends beyond individual patient outcomes, influencing public health strategies and policy-making. Successful clinical trials have the potential to transform standard of care practices, leading to improved health outcomes at the population level. For example, landmark trials in areas such as cardiovascular disease, oncology, and infectious diseases have resulted in paradigm shifts in treatment paradigms and substantial reductions in morbidity and mortality. Additionally, by elucidating the underlying mechanisms of diseases and therapeutic responses, clinical trials contribute to the development of personalized and precision medicine approaches, fostering tailored interventions that consider individual variations in genetics, lifestyle, and environmental factors.

The impact of clinical trials on medicine also underscores the importance of interdisciplinary collaboration and knowledge sharing. These research endeavors bring together a diverse array of stakeholders, including clinicians, scientists, regulatory authorities, industry partners, and most importantly, patients. Such collaborations foster a culture of innovation, driving transformative breakthroughs and accelerating the translation of scientific discoveries into tangible patient benefits. As technology and methodologies continue to evolve, clinical trials serve as incubators for cutting-edge approaches, including adaptive trial designs, real-world evidence integration, and digital health solutions.

In summary, the impact of clinical trials on medicine cannot be overstated. These rigorous investigations form the cornerstone of evidence-based medicine, shaping therapeutic landscapes, refining diagnostic modalities, and promoting health equity. As we navigate the complexities of modern healthcare, clinical trials remain an indispensable tool for addressing unmet medical needs, fostering scientific progress, and ultimately enhancing the well-being of individuals and communities.

Setting the Stage for Future Research

As we look to the future, it is crucial to consider how current clinical trials are shaping the landscape of healthcare research. By examining the outcomes and data yielded from these trials, researchers and medical professionals can identify areas for further investigation and development. This process sets the stage for future research endeavors that can potentially lead to breakthroughs in treatment and prevention strategies.

One key aspect of setting the stage for future research is the identification of emerging trends and patterns in clinical trial results. Analyzing the data collected from diverse participant groups enables researchers to pinpoint variations in treatment effectiveness based on factors such as age, gender, or underlying health conditions. These insights drive the formulation of targeted research questions aimed at understanding the underlying mechanisms behind these variations, ultimately informing the design of future clinical trials.

Furthermore, the dissemination of findings from completed clinical trials lays the groundwork for collaborative efforts among multidisciplinary teams. It fosters knowledge exchange and sparks discussions on refining existing methodologies or exploring innovative approaches to address persistent challenges in healthcare. This collaboration not only enhances the quality and scope of future research but also paves the way for interdisciplinary partnerships that can accelerate the translation of research findings into tangible clinical applications.

Additionally, as technological advancements continue to revolutionize healthcare, incorporating cutting-edge tools and methodologies into future clinical trials becomes imperative. From precision medicine to real-world evidence generation, embracing these innovations holds immense potential in refining the accuracy and efficiency of clinical research outcomes. Furthermore, leveraging digital platforms and telemedicine can enhance patient recruitment and engagement, thereby expanding the reach and inclusivity of future clinical trials.

In conclusion, setting the stage for future research in clinical trials demands a proactive and forward-thinking approach that integrates data-driven insights, collaboration, and the integration of emerging technologies. By harnessing the collective wisdom gained from current trials and embracing innovation, the healthcare community can foster an environment conducive to pioneering discoveries and transformative advances in patient care.

Phases of Clinical Trials

Introduction to the Phases of Clinical Trials

In the field of clinical research, the process of testing new medical interventions follows a systematic approach that is divided into phases. Each phase serves a specific purpose and has distinct objectives crucial to the overall success of the clinical trial. The overarching goal of the clinical trial phases is to systematically gather data on the safety and efficacy of the intervention being studied. Phase I trials primarily focus on evaluating the safety profile of the intervention in a small group of healthy volunteers or individuals with the disease under investigation. These trials aim to determine the maximum tolerated dose and identify potential side effects. Moving into Phase II, the primary objective shifts towards assessing the initial effectiveness of the intervention in a larger group of participants with the targeted health condition. This phase also provides further insights into the optimal dosage and potential risks. As the clinical trial progresses into Phase III, the key emphasis lies in confirming the effectiveness of the intervention, comparing it to existing standard treatments, and gathering more comprehensive safety data. Additionally, Phase III trials often involve a larger and more diverse participant population to ensure the generalizability of results. Finally, Phase IV, also known as post-marketing surveillance, occurs after regulatory approval and focuses on continuous assessment of the intervention's long-term safety and effectiveness in real-world settings. This phase plays a crucial role in monitoring rare adverse events and enhancing understanding of the intervention's broader impact. Understanding the distinct objectives and purposes of each phase is essential for researchers, clinicians, and regulatory authorities to collaboratively navigate the complex landscape of clinical trials and make informed decisions regarding the advancement of medical interventions.

Key Players in Clinical Trials

Clinical trials involve various key players who play crucial roles in ensuring the successful conduct of research while upholding ethical and regulatory standards. Understanding the responsibilities and contributions of these individuals and organizations is essential to appreciate the collaborative effort required in conducting clinical trials.

Role of the Food and Drug Administration (FDA): The FDA is a regulatory agency responsible for protecting public health by ensuring the safety, efficacy, and security of drugs, biological products, and medical devices. In the context of clinical trials, the FDA reviews and evaluates investigational new drug (IND) applications, investigational device exemptions (IDEs), and study protocols to assess the conduct and oversight of research involving human subjects. The FDA plays a critical role in safeguarding participants' rights and welfare, as well as in assessing the quality and integrity of the data generated from clinical trials. Additionally, the FDA provides guidance to Sponsors and investigators to help them understand and navigate the regulatory requirements for conducting clinical trials. This guidance can include advice on study design, data collection, and regulatory submissions.

Role of the Institutional Review Boards (IRB): IRBs are fundamental to the ethical oversight of clinical trials involving human subjects. These independent committees are composed of scientists, non-scientists, and community representatives who review, approve, and monitor research protocols to ensure that the rights, safety, and well-being of participants are protected. IRBs assess the risks and potential benefits of participation, evaluate the informed consent process, and conduct ongoing reviews to uphold ethical standards throughout the trial. IRBs bring diverse perspectives to the review process, ensuring that the research is scientifically valid and ethically sound. Moreover, they also provide education and guidance to researchers and the community about the ethical conduct of clinical research.

Role of the Sponsor/Contract Research Organization (CRO): The Sponsor or CRO assumes a significant role in driving the initiation and execution of clinical trials. Sponsors can be pharmaceutical companies, academic institutions, government agencies, or other organizations providing financial and organizational support for the research. They carry the ultimate responsibility for the trial's initiation, management, and oversight, including protocol development, regulatory submissions, and the establishment of quality assurance and data management systems. Contract Research Organizations (CROs) are external entities that Sponsors often engage to conduct various aspects of the trial, such as monitoring, data management, and statistical analysis, under the Sponsor's direction. Sponsors and CROs work closely with regulatory authorities to ensure compliance with regulations and to address any queries or concerns raised during the trial.

Role of the Principal Investigator (PI): The PI plays a pivotal role in conducting the trial at the investigational site. Alongside their medical or research expertise, the PI assumes responsibility for overseeing all aspects of the trial, including participant recruitment, protocol adherence, safety monitoring, and accurate data collection. As the individual ultimately accountable for the research's conduct, the PI ensures that the trial complies with regulatory requirements, maintains ethical standards, and upholds the scientific rigor essential to generating reliable and valid data. In addition to their scientific leadership, PIs also have administrative responsibilities, such as budget management and regulatory compliance, and serve as the primary point of contact for communication with the Sponsor, regulatory authorities, and the IRB at their site.

Role of the Clinical Research Coordinator (CRC): Clinical Research Coordinators are integral to the efficient and effective management of clinical trials. They are typically healthcare professionals or individuals who work with the Principal Investigator at the research site. CRCs have a strong background in clinical research and are responsible for coordinating various aspects of the trial, including participant recruitment, informed consent processes, data collection, and study visit coordination. Additionally, CRCs play a vital role in ensuring that the trial complies with the protocol, Good Clinical Practice (GCP) guidelines, and all applicable regulatory requirements while also maintaining the safety and well-being of participants. CRCs also facilitate the communication between the Sponsor/CRO, IRB, and the investigational site, ensuring that all parties are informed and aligned throughout the trial.

Role of the Clinical Research Associate (CRA): Clinical Research Associates, employed by the Sponsor or CRO, play a pivotal role in monitoring and overseeing the conduct of the clinical trial at investigational sites. They are typically responsible for site initiation, regular monitoring visits to assess protocol compliance and data quality, and ensuring that the trial is conducted in adherence to GCP guidelines and regulatory requirements. CRAs also maintain clear and effective communication with investigative site staff, supporting them in any protocol-related queries or issues that may arise during the course of the clinical trial. Their role also includes reviewing essential documents and records, ensuring that the site is prepared for regulatory inspections, and serving as a liaison between the site and

What Are Clinical Trials?

the Sponsor/CRO for any logistical or compliance-related matters.

In summary, the successful execution of clinical trials relies on the collaborative efforts of regulatory agencies, research institutions, Sponsors, investigators, and clinical research professionals. Each key player contributes to the ethical, regulatory, and scientific integrity of the trial, ultimately advancing medical knowledge and improving patient care.

By understanding the roles and responsibilities of these key players, stakeholders can appreciate the collective effort required to conduct clinical trials in an ethical and professional manner. Moreover, recognizing the significance of these key players can further drive collaboration, adherence to best practices, and the continual improvement of clinical trial processes to benefit patients and advance medical science.

Clinical Trial Design

Fundamentals of Trial Design

Clinical trial design is a crucial aspect of conducting valid and reliable research studies in the field of medicine. Fundamental principles such as randomization, blinding, and placebo control play pivotal roles in minimizing bias and ensuring the integrity of trial results. Randomization is the process of assigning participants to treatment or control groups by chance, rather than by choice or preference. This method helps to distribute both known and unknown confounding factors equally between groups, thus reducing the potential for systematic errors and enhancing the internal validity of the study. Blinding, also known as masking, involves withholding specific information from participants, investigators, or both, to prevent conscious or subconscious biases that could influence the outcome assessment. By maintaining blinding, the impact of subjective influences on participant-reported outcomes and investigator-assessed endpoints can be mitigated, supporting the objectivity of the trial findings. Furthermore, placebo control, where applicable, serves as a valuable tool in distinguishing the true effects of a medical intervention from those that may arise due to psychological or contextual factors. Implementing these fundamental principles not only upholds the scientific rigor of clinical trials but also promotes transparency and trust within the medical community and among patients. As such, a comprehensive understanding of these foundational elements is essential for researchers, clinicians, and stakeholders involved in the design and implementation of clinical trials.

Selection of Control and Treatment Groups

What Are Clinical Trials?

The selection of control and treatment groups is an aspect of clinical trial design, as it directly influences the validity and reliability of the study results. In order to compare the effects of a new treatment with existing standard care or placebo, control and treatment groups must be carefully designed and assigned. The control group serves as the benchmark for comparison, receiving either no treatment, standard treatment, or a placebo, while the treatment group receives the experimental intervention under investigation.

When selecting control and treatment groups, researchers must consider various factors to ensure the fairness and accuracy of the comparisons. Random assignment is often employed to allocate participants to either the control or treatment group, minimizing the potential for bias and ensuring that participants have an equal chance of being in either group. Additionally, researchers must carefully consider the characteristics of the study population to ensure that both groups are representative and comparable in terms of demographics, disease severity, and other relevant variables.

Another important consideration is blinding, where participants, investigators, and data analysts are kept unaware of the group assignments to reduce the influence of biases on the results. Blinding can take the form of single-blind, double-blind, or even triple-blind designs, depending on the nature of the intervention and the study objectives.

Furthermore, the proper choice of control group is crucial in determining the efficacy and safety of the new treatment. For example, in comparative drug trials, the use of an active control group (receiving an established treatment) allows for direct comparison with the investigational treatment, whereas a placebo control group provides a baseline for evaluating the true effect of the intervention. Careful consideration is also given to the timing and duration of the control and treatment interventions, ensuring consistent and meaningful comparisons between the groups over the course of the trial.

Moreover, ethical considerations play a significant role in the selection of control and treatment groups. Researchers must uphold the principles of beneficence and non-maleficence, ensuring that participants in the control group receive an appropriate standard of care and are not exposed to unnecessary risks. Equitable access to potential benefits and protection from harm are paramount concerns in the design and implementation of clinical trials.

In summary, the selection of control and treatment groups is a multifaceted process that requires careful attention to scientific, ethical, and logistical considerations. By thoughtfully designing these groups, researchers can enhance the quality and validity of clinical trial outcomes, ultimately contributing to the advancement of medical knowledge and the improvement of patient care.

Endpoints and Outcome Measures

In clinical trial design, the selection of appropriate endpoints and outcome measures is crucial for evaluating the safety and efficacy of a new intervention. Endpoints refer to the specific events or outcomes that are measured to determine the effect of the treatment, while outcome measures are the actual instruments or methods used to assess these endpoints.

When considering endpoints, researchers must identify outcomes that are not only clinically meaningful but also feasible to measure within the confines of the trial. This involves careful consideration of both primary and secondary endpoints. The primary endpoint is the key outcome that the trial is designed to measure, directly reflecting the drug's effect on patients' health. Secondary endpoints provide additional valuable information and can support the findings related to the primary endpoint.

In the selection of outcome measures, it is important to use well-validated and reliable tools to accurately capture the intended endpoints. These measures can take various forms, including clinical assessments, laboratory tests, patient-reported outcomes, and radiological imaging. The choice of outcome measures should align with the specific objectives of the trial and be sensitive enough to detect meaningful differences between the treatment and control groups.

Moreover, the timing and frequency of measuring endpoints and outcome measures play a critical role in ensuring the trial's success. Establishing clear guidelines for when and how these assessments will be conducted helps maintain consistency and uniformity across the trial, reducing potential biases and ensuring the reliability of the data collected.

Throughout the process of selecting endpoints and outcome measures, the input of multidisciplinary experts, including clinicians, statisticians, and regulatory authorities, is invaluable. Collaboration among these stakeholders helps ensure that the chosen endpoints and measures are not only scientifically sound but also align with regulatory requirements and the practical realities of implementing the trial.

Overall, thoughtful consideration of endpoints and outcome measures is essential to the design and execution of a successful clinical trial. By choosing endpoints that accurately reflect the impact of the intervention and using validated outcome measures, researchers can confidently evaluate the treatment's effectiveness and safety, ultimately advancing medical knowledge and improving patient care.

Informed Consent Process

Foundations of Informed Consent

Informed consent is an important component of ethical clinical research, rooted in both philosophical and legal principles. At its core, informed consent respects individuals' autonomy and right to make decisions about their participation in medical research. Philosophically, informed consent reflects the fundamental ethical principle of respect for persons, as outlined in the Belmont Report. This principle recognizes individuals as autonomous agents capable of making independent decisions with regard to their own well-being. From a legal perspective, the requirement for informed consent has been established through landmark court cases and statutes that underscore the importance of protecting participants' rights and ensuring their voluntary participation. By understanding the philosophical and legal underpinnings of informed consent, researchers and healthcare professionals can appreciate its significance in upholding participants' autonomy and promoting ethical conduct. Moreover, a strong foundation in informed consent is essential for fostering trust between researchers and participants, ultimately contributing to the advancement of medical knowledge and improved patient care.

Procedures and Documentation

The procedures for obtaining informed consent involve multiple steps to ensure that potential participants fully understand the nature of the clinical trial and the implications of their participation. Key elements of this process include the disclosure of relevant information, the competency of the individual providing consent, and the documentation of the consent. The first step in the process is the disclosure of relevant information, which includes details regarding the purpose, procedures, benefits, potential risks, and alternatives to participation in the clinical trial. This information should be presented in a clear, understandable manner, free from any coercion or undue influence.

Following the disclosure of information, the potential participant must demonstrate their understanding of the provided details. This may involve an assessment of their comprehension, ensuring that they are capable of making an informed decision. This assessment is crucial in determining the participant's competence to provide consent.

Once the individual has demonstrated an understanding of the information and is deemed competent to provide consent, the actual consent is documented. This documentation typically takes the form of a written consent form, signed by the participant or their legally authorized representative. The consent form outlines the details of the trial and serves as evidence that the participant has voluntarily agreed to take part in the study.

Furthermore, the documentation process also involves providing a copy of the consent form to the participant, offering them the opportunity to retain a record of their agreement. In certain cases, the use of audio-visual recordings may supplement the written documentation, especially when dealing with complex procedures or vulnerable populations. These recordings can serve as additional proofs of the consent process, enhancing transparency and accountability.

Overall, the procedures and documentation associated with informed consent are critical components of ethical clinical research. They serve to protect the rights and well-being of research participants, uphold the integrity of the research process, and ensure compliance with regulatory requirements.

Challenges and Solutions in Informed Consent

Informed consent within clinical trials is a critical process, yet it can present various challenges that require careful consideration and proactive solutions. One fundamental challenge is ensuring that participants fully comprehend the information provided to them regarding the trial, its potential risks, and benefits. This may be especially complex if the participant has limited health literacy or if English is not their primary language. To address this challenge, it is essential to incorporate clear and concise language in the informed consent documents, to provide the informed consent in the subject native language, or to provide interpreter services when necessary.

Another significant challenge in the informed consent process is obtaining consent from vulnerable populations such as children or individuals with cognitive impairments. Balancing the need for research within these populations while also protecting their rights and well-being requires innovative solutions. For instance, utilizing age-appropriate educational materials when obtaining assent from minors, or employing advanced decision-making tools when working with individuals who may have difficulty comprehending the complexities of the trial.

Additionally, maintaining ongoing communication with participants throughout the trial presents a continuous challenge. Participants may encounter unforeseen changes in their health status or experience unanticipated side effects, which could influence their willingness to continue participating. Regular contact and support from the site research team are vital in addressing these concerns and promoting retention in the trial.

Furthermore, ensuring that the consent process remains ethically sound and complies with evolving regulatory standards poses an ongoing challenge. Research institutions must adapt to updated guidelines and ensure that all staff involved in obtaining consent receive proper training in ethical considerations. Furthermore, the rise of digital platforms brings new challenges related to obtaining electronic consent; this necessitates robust cybersecurity measures and verifiable digital signatures to maintain the integrity of the consent process.

To address these challenges, collaborative efforts involving researchers, ethicists, clinicians, and community representatives are crucial. By engaging in dialogues and sharing best practices, the research community can develop innovative solutions and continuously improve the informed consent process, thereby upholding the principles of autonomy, beneficence, and justice in clinical research.

Recruitment and Enrollment

Strategies for Effective Recruitment

Recruiting participants for clinical trials is an essential element of the research process, as the success of a trial often hinges on the ability to enroll a diverse and representative sample of participants. One effective strategy for recruitment is the utilization of online advertisement. This method allows researchers to reach a large audience quickly through various digital platforms, such as social media, search engines, and targeted websites. By crafting compelling and informative advertisements, researchers can attract individuals who may be interested in participating in the clinical trial.

Another valuable method for recruitment is community engagement. This involves partnering with local organizations, healthcare providers, and community leaders to raise awareness about the clinical trial and its potential impact. Community events, seminars, and outreach programs can effectively disseminate information about the trial, reaching individuals who might not have otherwise been aware of the opportunity to participate. Building trust within the community is essential for successful recruitment, and establishing strong relationships with community stakeholders can enhance the credibility and legitimacy of the trial.

Additionally, clinician referrals provide a targeted approach to recruitment, as healthcare professionals can directly identify and refer eligible patients to the trial. Physicians, nurses, and other healthcare providers play a crucial role in informing their patients about the opportunity to participate in a clinical trial. Their expertise and guidance can help potential participants understand the significance of the research and feel confident in their decision to enroll.

In summary, employing a multifaceted approach to recruitment, including online advertising, community engagement, and clinician referrals, can enhance the effectiveness of participant recruitment for clinical trials. By leveraging these strategies, researchers can increase the likelihood of enrolling a diverse and representative cohort, contributing to the overall success and validity of the trial.

Eligibility Criteria and Participant Selection

Establishing clear and specific eligibility criteria is essential to ensure that the participants enrolled in the trial are representative of the target patient population. This section will delve into the various aspects of eligibility criteria and participant selection, addressing their significance and impact on the integrity of clinical trial results. Firstly, defining precise inclusion and exclusion criteria is fundamental in identifying individuals who meet the desired characteristics for the study while excluding those with factors that could potentially skew the results. Factors such as age, gender, medical history, and specific health conditions must be carefully considered when formulating these criteria. Additionally, accounting for demographic diversity within the eligible participant pool is imperative to ensure that the trial results can be applied to a broader population. Furthermore, the process of participant selection involves careful consideration of ethical principles to safeguard participants' well-being. It is critical to adhere to ethical guidelines to prevent any form of bias or discrimination during the selection process, ensuring fair and equitable participation opportunities. In addition to ethical considerations, practical aspects such as geographical location, accessibility to healthcare facilities, and availability of resources may also impact participant selection. Therefore, careful planning and assessment are necessary to address these logistical challenges. Moreover, engaging healthcare professionals and clinical investigators to aid in the identification and referral of potential participants can streamline the selection process and enhance the likelihood of enrolling suitable candidates. Furthermore, fostering transparent communication about the trial's objectives, potential benefits, and risks is essential to facilitate informed decision-making among prospective participants. Engaging in open dialogue with individuals considering participation can help manage their expectations and clarify any inquiries regarding the trial. Ultimately, by meticulously evaluating eligibility criteria and executing a comprehensive participant selection process, clinical trials can assemble a diverse and representative cohort that aligns with the study's objectives, thereby enhancing the validity and generalizability of the findings.

Challenges in Recruitment and Solutions

Recruiting participants for clinical trials can be a complex and challenging task, often posing significant obstacles for researchers. One of the primary challenges is the reluctance of potential participants to engage in clinical trials due to fear or skepticism about the research process. Additionally, reaching out to diverse and underrepresented populations can be difficult, leading to limited diversity in the participant pool, which may impact the generalizability of study results. Furthermore, competition with other ongoing trials for recruiting participants also presents a hurdle. To address these challenges, several solutions can be implemented. Firstly, it is crucial to establish clear and transparent communication channels to educate and inform the public about the importance and benefits of clinical trials. This can help dispel misconceptions and build trust within the community. Collaborating with community organizations and healthcare providers can also aid in reaching a wider demographic and fostering relationships based on mutual respect and understanding. Moreover, utilizing targeted marketing strategies through various media channels can help raise awareness and attract potential participants. Developing personalized recruitment approaches that consider the cultural and linguistic needs of different populations can further enhance outreach efforts. In addition, offering incentives and compensation for participation can incentivize individuals to consider enrolling in clinical trials. It's also vital to streamline the enrollment process, ensuring that it is convenient and accessible for potential participants. Incorporating digital platforms and telemedicine options can facilitate remote participation, making it easier for individuals from diverse geographic locations to take part in the research as well. By overcoming these challenges through proactive and innovative solutions, researchers can improve participant recruitment, thereby enhancing the overall quality and impact of clinical trials.

Conducting Clinical Trials

Trial Operations and Management

Clinical trial operations and management encompass the intricate coordination of various essential components to ensure the seamless execution of the trial. At the forefront is diligent site management, involving the oversight and supervision of all activities conducted at the trial sites. This encompasses a spectrum of responsibilities, including but not limited to ensuring compliance with protocol requirements, overseeing participant recruitment and retention efforts, managing investigational product storage and handling, and maintaining accurate and comprehensive records of all trial-related activities.

An integral aspect of trial operations and management relates to the coordination between diverse stakeholders involved in the clinical trial process. This involves establishing effective lines of communication and collaboration between Sponsors, investigators, clinical research coordinators, institutional review boards, ethics committees, and regulatory authorities. Facilitating transparent and efficient information exchange among these stakeholders is imperative for fostering a conducive environment that promotes adherence to ethical and regulatory standards.

Moreover, successful trial operations and management necessitate a robust infrastructure to support the collection, analysis, and dissemination of data. Timely and accurate data capture and reporting are critical to deriving meaningful insights and conclusions. Furthermore, this requires the implementation of stringent quality control measures to uphold the reliability and integrity of the data collected throughout the trial.

In addition to overseeing the daily operations of clinical trials, proactive risk management strategies play a pivotal role in mitigating potential challenges and ensuring the smooth progression of the trial. This encompasses the implementation of contingency plans and adaptive measures to address unforeseen circumstances or deviations from the planned course of action. Through proactive planning and vigilant oversight, clinical trial operations and management aim to uphold the highest standards of quality, integrity, and participant safety while advancing scientific knowledge and medical innovation.

Monitoring and Quality Control

Clinical trials require stringent monitoring and quality control measures to ensure the integrity of the data and the safety of the participants. In this section, we will delve into the crucial aspects of monitoring and maintaining quality throughout the trial process. Monitoring in clinical trials involves the oversight of trial conduct, data collection, and adherence to the protocol. This is typically carried out by appointed individuals or committees who are responsible for regularly reviewing the progress of the trial and ensuring that it is conducted in compliance with Good Clinical Practice (GCP) guidelines and relevant regulations. Quality control, on the other hand, focuses on implementing measures to guarantee the accuracy, reliability, and consistency of the collected data. This includes validation of instruments, regular calibration of equipment, and meticulous documentation of all procedures. It is imperative for clinical trial Sponsors to establish robust quality control processes to minimize errors and maintain the credibility of the trial results. Effective monitoring and quality control not only contribute to the success of the trial but also safeguard the well-being of the participants. By continuously assessing the conduct and data of the trial, potential issues can be promptly identified and addressed. Proactive monitoring enables early detection of any deviations from the protocol, ensuring that corrective actions can be taken swiftly, thus safeguarding the trial's validity and the well-being of its participants. In addition, robust quality control measures help to ensure that the data collected is accurate and reliable, providing a solid foundation for analysis and interpretation. As technology continues to advance, innovative methods for monitoring and quality control in clinical trials have emerged, offering real-time data monitoring, risk-based monitoring approaches, and sophisticated data analytics tools. Embracing these advancements can enhance the efficiency and accuracy of trial oversight, ultimately leading to better outcomes for both researchers and participants. It is worth noting that while stringent monitoring and quality control measures are essential, they should be implemented judiciously, taking into consideration the specific requirements of the trial and the ethical considerations associated with human subject research. Balancing these factors is paramount to upholding the scientific rigor and ethical standards crucial to the success and integrity of clinical trials.

Addressing Challenges and Adaptations

Clinical trials are complex endeavors that often encounter various challenges and require the ability to adapt to unforeseen circumstances. In this section, we will delve into the key strategies for addressing challenges and making necessary adaptations during the course of conducting clinical trials.

One of the primary challenges in clinical trials is patient recruitment and retention. Addressing this challenge involves developing innovative strategies to enhance participant engagement and compliance with study protocols. This may include leveraging digital technologies for remote monitoring and providing incentives for participation in the trial.

Another common hurdle is managing protocol deviations or unexpected adverse events. It is essential to have robust oversight mechanisms in place to promptly identify and address such issues. Additionally, maintaining open communication with regulatory authorities and institutional review boards is critical when implementing necessary adaptations to the study protocol in response to emerging challenges.

Furthermore, ensuring the quality and integrity of data throughout the trial is paramount. This involves proactive measures such as implementing thorough training for site staff, employing centralized monitoring techniques, and utilizing electronic data capture systems to minimize errors and discrepancies.

In addition to these operational challenges, clinical trials may also face external factors such as changes in regulatory requirements or advancements in standard of care. Effective adaptation to such external influences requires a comprehensive understanding of the evolving landscape and proactive collaboration with relevant stakeholders.

Moreover, it is crucial to maintain flexibility in resource allocation and budget management to accommodate unexpected needs or adjustments in trial conduct. This necessitates ongoing assessment of resource utilization and rigorous risk management strategies to ensure effective adaptation without compromising the integrity of the trial.

Ultimately, addressing challenges and making adaptations in clinical trials demands a multidisciplinary approach that integrates expertise from clinical research, regulatory affairs, project management, and data analytics. By fostering a culture of continuous improvement and responsiveness, clinical trial teams can navigate obstacles with agility and uphold the scientific rigor and ethical principles of the study.

Data Analysis and Interpretation

Statistical Techniques and Tools

In the realm of clinical trials, statistical techniques and tools play a crucial role in analyzing data to derive meaningful insights. Various statistical models are employed to evaluate the efficacy and safety of interventions, assess patient outcomes, and make informed decisions about potential treatments. These models include but are not limited to linear regression, logistic regression, survival analysis, and mixed-effects models. Each model serves a specific purpose and is selected based on the nature of the data and the research questions being addressed. Furthermore, the role of software and automation in statistical analysis cannot be overstated. With the increasing complexity and volume of clinical trial data, specialized software such as SAS, R, or Python are utilized for advanced data manipulation, visualization, and statistical modeling. These tools enable researchers to perform intricate analyses with accuracy and efficiency. Automation also plays a significant role in streamlining repetitive tasks, ensuring consistency, and reducing human error in data processing and statistical computations. As technology continues to advance, the integration of artificial intelligence and machine learning algorithms in statistical analysis holds great promise for revolutionizing data interpretation within clinical contexts. Overall, understanding and leveraging statistical techniques and tools are paramount in ensuring the quality and reliability of findings derived from clinical trial data.

Interpreting Data Within Clinical Contexts

Interpreting clinical trial data within the context of healthcare is a critical step in deriving meaningful conclusions and insights. It involves a comprehensive understanding of the specific medical conditions under study, treatment modalities, and patient demographics. Interpreting data within clinical contexts necessitates a nuanced approach that considers not only statistical significance but also clinical relevance. Healthcare professionals play a vital role in this process, leveraging their expertise to contextualize and understand the implications of the data. Moreover, it is essential to collaborate closely with medical practitioners to gain valuable insights into the real-world patient scenarios, thereby enriching the interpretation of clinical trial data. Understanding the clinical significance of statistical findings is imperative in making informed decisions about treatment efficacy and safety. Additionally, factors such as comorbidities, concomitant medications, and patient compliance must be carefully considered when interpreting data within clinical contexts. This stage holds significant importance in ensuring that the results obtained from the clinical trials are translatable into meaningful advancements in patient care. Furthermore, the interpretation process should also encompass the potential impact of the study outcomes on current medical practices and guidelines. By bridging the gap between statistical findings and clinical implications, researchers can contribute to the evolution of evidence-based healthcare practices and improve patient outcomes.

Presenting Results to Stakeholders

Presenting the results of clinical trials to stakeholders is a significant part of the research process. Effective communication of findings ensures that the significance of the study and its potential impact are clearly conveyed to all relevant parties. This section will explore the key considerations and best practices for presenting clinical trial results to stakeholders.

1. Tailoring Communication: When presenting results to stakeholders, it is essential to tailor the communication to suit the audience. Stakeholders may include researchers, healthcare professionals, regulatory authorities, patients, and the wider public. Each group has distinct levels of expertise and specific information needs. Therefore, the presentation of results should be adapted to ensure that it is comprehensible and relevant to each stakeholder group.

2. Accuracy and Transparency: An emphasis on accuracy and transparency is crucial in presenting clinical trial results. Stakeholders rely on the integrity of the data and the methods used for analysis. It is imperative to provide a clear and comprehensive overview of the study design, methodology, and statistical analyses employed. Any limitations or potential biases in the data should also be clearly communicated to ensure a complete understanding of the findings.

3. Visual Representations: Utilizing visual representations such as graphs, charts, figures, and tables can significantly enhance the comprehension of complex data sets. Visual aids offer a succinct and compelling way to present key findings, trends, and comparisons. However, it is essential to ensure that visual representations are accurately labeled, easy to interpret, and do not distort the underlying data.

4. Clinical Relevance: Presenting results within the clinical context is vital for stakeholders to grasp the implications of the findings. It is important to articulate the real-world relevance of the results, illustrating how they may impact patient care, treatment guidelines, or future research directions. Providing concrete examples and case studies can help stakeholders

appreciate the practical applications of the study outcomes.

5. Interactive Engagement: Engaging stakeholders in a dialogue rather than delivering a unidirectional presentation fosters a more collaborative and informed exchange of information. Opportunities for questions, discussions, and feedback serve to clarify any uncertainties and demonstrate a commitment to open communication. Furthermore, soliciting input from stakeholders can aid in identifying areas for further exploration or refinement of the research findings.

By adhering to these principles and practices, researchers and Sponsors can effectively present the results of clinical trials to stakeholders in a manner that is informative, transparent, and engaging. Such presentations play a pivotal role in shaping the understanding and acceptance of the research outcomes and ultimately contribute to advancements in healthcare and medical knowledge.

Ethical and Regulatory Considerations

Foundational Ethics in Clinical Research

Ethical principles such as respect for people, beneficence, and justice form the cornerstone of clinical research. Respect for people acknowledges individuals' autonomy and emphasizes the importance of obtaining informed consent from participants before their inclusion in a clinical trial. This principle also underscores the need to protect the privacy and confidentiality of participants. Beneficence underscores the ethical imperative to maximize benefits and minimize potential harms to participants in clinical research. Researchers must ensure that the potential risks are justified by the anticipated benefits and take all steps necessary to optimize the well-being of participants. In addition, justice demands that the selection of research subjects be fair and that the burdens and benefits of research be distributed equitably. It also extends to ensuring that vulnerable populations are not disproportionately represented in clinical trials and have equal access to the potential benefits of research. These three ethical principles serve as the moral compass guiding all aspects of clinical research, from study design to participant recruitment and retention, data collection, and dissemination of results. By upholding these principles, researchers, Sponsors, and institutional review boards (IRBs) can ensure the integrity and trustworthiness of clinical research, ultimately advancing medical knowledge and benefiting society at large.

Regulatory Frameworks and Compliance

Regulatory frameworks and compliance are integral components of clinical trials, ensuring the protection of participant rights and the integrity of research data. Regulatory bodies such as the Food and Drug

Administration (FDA) in the United States and the European Medicines Agency (EMA) in Europe play a crucial role in overseeing the conduct of clinical trials. These agencies establish guidelines and regulations that govern various aspects of clinical research, including study design, participant recruitment, informed consent processes, and safety monitoring. By adhering to these regulations, researchers and Sponsors uphold the ethical standards and scientific rigor essential to conducting valid and reliable clinical trials.

Compliance with regulatory requirements involves meticulous attention to detail at every stage of the trial. Researchers must thoroughly document their adherence to the protocol and procedural guidelines to demonstrate compliance with regulatory standards. This documentation includes obtaining approval from institutional review boards (IRBs) or independent ethics committees, maintaining accurate records of participant enrollment and adverse events, and submitting timely and comprehensive reports to regulatory authorities.

In addition to adhering to regulatory directives, achieving compliance also demands a deep understanding of the specific regulatory landscape governing the geographical location where the clinical trial is being conducted. Each country may have its own set of regulations and oversight mechanisms, which necessitates careful navigation for successful compliance. This complexity underscores the importance of engaging experts in regulatory affairs and seeking legal counsel to ensure full compliance with all applicable laws and regulations.

Furthermore, compliance with regulatory frameworks extends beyond the immediate operational aspects of the trial and encompasses broader considerations such as data privacy protection and transparency. With the proliferation of electronic data capture systems and the increasing digitalization of clinical trials, ensuring the security and confidentiality of participant information has become a critical regulatory concern. Researchers and Sponsors must implement robust data management practices in compliance with data protection regulations to safeguard participant privacy and maintain the integrity of trial data.

Ultimately, the meticulous observance of regulatory frameworks and compliance requirements is not just a legal obligation; it is a fundamental ethical imperative in conducting clinical trials. By prioritizing adherence to regulatory standards, researchers and Sponsors uphold the trust of participants, healthcare providers, and regulatory agencies, thereby contributing to the advancement of safe and effective medical interventions for the benefit of society.

Contemporary Issues and Case Studies

In the ever-evolving landscape of clinical research, the identification and examination of contemporary ethical and regulatory issues are imperative to ensuring the integrity of clinical trials. This section delves into a comprehensive exploration of pertinent case studies and current issues that have significant implications for the ethical conduct and governance of clinical trials.

One of the prominent contemporary issues in clinical research involves the utilization of big data and the challenges associated with protecting participant privacy and confidentiality. With the rapid advancements in technology and the utilization of electronic health records, the collection and analysis of extensive datasets has become commonplace in clinical trials. However, safeguarding the privacy of participants and maintaining the confidentiality of their personal information poses complex ethical dilemmas that demand careful consideration.

Furthermore, the globalization of clinical trials has emerged as a critical concern in the regulatory and ethical realms. The conduct of trials across diverse geographic regions introduces multifaceted challenges related to varying cultural norms, healthcare systems, and socio-economic factors. Addressing these disparities while upholding ethical standards and ensuring participant welfare requires a nuanced understanding of the unique complexities inherent in international clinical research.

The integration of innovative therapies and interventions in clinical trials necessitates a meticulous examination of ethical considerations and regulatory frameworks. By delving into compelling case studies, this section elucidates the ethical complexities inherent in experimental treatments, such as gene therapy and immunotherapy. These groundbreaking approaches present unprecedented ethical challenges pertaining to risk-benefit assessments, informed consent, and equitable access to novel treatments, underscoring the critical importance of aligning advancements in medical science with robust ethical oversight.

Additionally, the emergence of social media and digital platforms as tools for patient recruitment and engagement has reshaped the dynamics of clinical research. Exploring the responsible utilization of these technologies and mitigating potential ethical pitfalls is essential in maintaining the trustworthiness and reliability of trial results.

Through the in-depth examination of contemporary ethical and regulatory issues, coupled with illuminating case studies, this section aims to provide readers with a nuanced understanding of the multifaceted considerations underpinning the ethical conduct of clinical trials. By engaging with these crucial topics, researchers, ethicists, and regulatory authorities can collaboratively contribute to the ongoing evolution and enhancement of ethical practices in the realm of clinical research.

Benefits and Risks of Participation

Evaluating the Advantages of Participation

Participating in clinical trials offers individuals a unique opportunity to potentially access new treatments and be at the forefront of medical advancements. Clinical trials provide participants with early access to innovative therapies that may not yet be widely available, allowing them to receive leading-edge medical care before it becomes accessible to the general public. By enrolling in these trials, individuals can gain access to novel medications, procedures, or devices that have the potential to improve their health outcomes or even extend their lives. Furthermore, participation in clinical trials can also offer a sense of personal satisfaction by contributing to the progress of medical research. Contributing to the development of new treatments and interventions allows participants to play an active role in advancing healthcare for themselves and future generations. The knowledge gained from individuals who participate in clinical trials is invaluable in furthering scientific understanding and paving the way for improved healthcare practices. Thus, the decision to participate in a clinical trial should be carefully considered, as it presents the potential for both personal health benefits and broader contributions to medical science.

Understanding Potential Risks and Discomforts

One of the crucial aspects of clinical trial participation is to have a comprehensive understanding of the potential risks and discomforts associated with the process. Participants need to be informed about the various risks that may arise during the course of a clinical trial, ranging from mild discomforts to more serious adverse reactions.

In any clinical trial, there are inherent risks involved due to the experimental nature of the interventions being tested. These can include the possibility of experiencing known side effects of the investigational treatment, as well as the chance of unforeseen adverse events. It is essential for prospective participants to recognize that these risks are an inherent part of the scientific process and are carefully monitored throughout the trial.

Furthermore, it's important to acknowledge that participation in a clinical trial may also pose inconveniences and discomforts. These could range from frequent visits to the trial site for assessments and follow-ups to potential limitations on certain activities or treatments. Patients should be made aware of these potential inconveniences beforehand to make an informed decision about their participation.

To ensure that participants are well-informed about the potential risks and discomforts, researchers and healthcare professionals have a responsibility to openly communicate this information in a transparent and understandable manner. This involves providing detailed explanations of the possible risks and discomforts, as well as addressing any concerns or questions that the participants may have. In addition, participants should be educated about the measures in place to minimize and manage these risks and discomforts.

It is also crucial for participants to understand that they have the right to withdraw from the clinical trial at any time if they experience unexpected discomfort or if they no longer wish to continue their participation. This emphasizes the importance of ongoing communication between participants and the research team to ensure that any emerging issues are identified and responded to promptly.

By gaining a comprehensive understanding of the potential risks and discomforts associated with clinical trial participation, individuals are better equipped to make informed decisions about their involvement. Ultimately, ensuring that participants are fully aware of these aspects contributes to safeguarding their well-being and upholding the ethical standards of clinical research.

Balancing Benefits Against Risks for Informed Decisions

In the complex landscape of clinical trials, it is essential for potential participants to carefully consider and weigh the benefits against the risks before making an informed decision. One of the primary aspects to evaluate when considering participation in a clinical trial is the potential health benefits that could result from access to innovative treatments or contributing to medical advancements. It is important for individuals to understand the nature of the condition being studied and the likelihood of the trial providing a beneficial outcome in their specific case.

It is also important to recognize that informed decision-making in clinical trials extends beyond personal considerations. Participants should be encouraged to evaluate the broader impact of their involvement, including the potential contributions to scientific knowledge and the advancement of medical treatments for future generations. Recognizing the altruistic aspect of participation can provide a deeper sense of purpose and fulfillment to those considering enrollment in a clinical trial.

Ultimately, the process of balancing benefits against risks for informed decisions demands careful reflection and a comprehensive understanding of the trial's implications. As individuals navigate this pivotal decision-making process, they are encouraged to seek support from their trusted healthcare providers, research team, and loved ones to ensure that their choices align with their best interests. By fostering an environment of informed decision-making, participants can approach clinical trial participation with confidence and clarity, taking active roles in shaping the future of medical research while prioritizing their well-being.

What Are Clinical Trials?

Conclusion

Summary of Key Findings

In summarizing the key findings from previous chapters, it is essential to recap the main objectives, methodologies, and discoveries that have been elucidated throughout this comprehensive exploration of clinical trials. The initial chapters delved into the purpose of clinical trials, highlighting their crucial role in advancing medical science and improving patient care. As we progressed through the subsequent sections, the different phases of clinical trials were meticulously examined, explicating the distinct purposes and methodologies employed in each phase, thereby emphasizing the progression of evidence-based research. Furthermore, the key participants in clinical trials, encompassing the roles and responsibilities of researchers, Sponsors, and participants, were thoroughly explained, shedding light on the collaborative efforts required to ensure the success and integrity of clinical trials. The chapter on clinical trial design provided valuable insight into the intricacies of designing a robust and effective trial, considering factors such as study endpoints, randomization, and blinding. One of the most pivotal aspects, the informed consent process, was given substantial attention, underlining the ethical imperative of ensuring participants' understanding and autonomy in decision-making. Moreover, the challenges and strategies related to recruitment and enrollment were expounded upon, accentuating the significance of diverse and representative participant populations to enhance the generalizability of trial findings. The subsequent chapters scrutinized the meticulous processes involved in conducting clinical trials, including data collection, monitoring, and ensuring adherence to protocols, all of which are fundamental for generating reliable and valid results. Through detailed discussions on data analysis and interpretation, readers were apprised of the intricate statistical methodologies employed to derive meaningful conclusions from trial data. In addition, ethical and regulatory considerations were delineated in depth, emphasizing the paramount necessity of adhering to ethical guidelines and regulatory protocols to safeguard participants' rights and ensure the integrity of research outcomes. The multifaceted discussion on the benefits and risks of participation provided nuanced insights into the implications and responsibilities associated with participating in clinical trials, thus equipping readers with a comprehensive understanding of the complexities inherent in this realm. Hence, by summarizing these key findings, we underscore the intricate tapestry of knowledge and insights woven throughout this book, setting the stage for an informed reflection on the future directions of clinical trials.

Future Directions in Clinical Trials

As the field of clinical trials continues to evolve, several future directions are poised to shape its trajectory. One of the most prominent areas of development lies in the integration of digital health technologies into clinical trial protocols. Advancements in wearable devices and mobile health applications offer the potential to revolutionize data collection and patient monitoring, ultimately enhancing the accuracy and efficiency of clinical trials. Also, the utilization of adaptive trial designs is gaining momentum, enabling real-time modifications based on accumulating data, which can optimize resource utilization and shorten trial durations.

Another pivotal aspect of future clinical trials pertains to precision medicine, wherein treatments are tailored to individual genetic, environmental, and lifestyle factors. Such personalized approaches hold promise for improved treatment outcomes and reduced adverse events. Furthermore, the incorporation of electronic patient-reported outcomes (ePROs) and patient-centric trial design will be instrumental in ensuring that clinical trials align with the priorities and experiences of the individuals they aim to benefit.

In order to address issues of diversity and inclusion, future clinical trials will be required to place greater emphasis on recruiting diverse participant populations to better reflect the demographics of the target patient groups. This commitment to diversity not only fosters equitable access to innovative therapies but also ensures the generalizability of trial results across different demographic subgroups.

Moreover, the evolution of regulatory frameworks and ethical considerations will play a vital role in shaping the landscape of clinical trials. Streamlined regulatory processes and novel ethical guidelines can facilitate the timely and responsible conduct of trials while upholding participant safety and autonomy. Embracing transparency and open science practices is another noteworthy trend, promoting data sharing, collaborative research, and reproducibility of findings to fortify the robustness of clinical evidence.

The convergence of these future directions holds the potential to propel clinical trials into an era characterized by enhanced efficiency, inclusivity, and patient-centeredness, thereby advancing the collective pursuit of improving healthcare outcomes and expanding the frontiers of medical knowledge.

About the Author

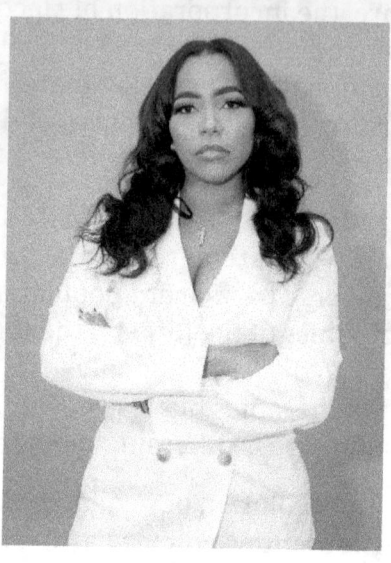

Dr. Chardae Rodgers-Gamble is the CEO and owner of CR Clinical. Dr. Rodgers-Gamble is a Clinical Operations Professional with over 13 years of experience in the clinical research industry. She has worked as a Clinical Research Associate, Clinical Trial Manager, Clinical Project Manager, and Clinical Project Lead along with providing pharmaceutical companies and CROs with full clinical research services. She has worked in multiple indications of clinical research such as gynecology, infectious disease, rare disease, oncology, neurology, cardiology, endocrinology, gastroenterology, pulmonary, ophthalmology, dermatology, orthopedic, and many other therapeutic areas. Dr. Rodgers-Gamble has been featured in the Women Leaders Magazine as the "20 Most Inspiring Women Leaders of 2022 and in Aspioneer as "The Trailblazer, Women Leaders of 2023" for her excellent work in clinical research as the CEO of CR Clinical. Most recently, Marquis Who's Who honored Dr. Chardae Rodgers-Gamble in 2024, for her Expertise in Clinical Research and Pharmaceuticals.

What Are Clinical Trials?

CR Clinical is a full-service Contract Research Organization (CRO). We provide a comprehensive solution for all clinical research needs along with offering outsourcing services to meet the evolving demands of the industry. We establish strategic partnerships with leading pharmaceutical, biotech, medical device corporations, Contract Research Organizations (CROs), & individual professionals to conduct clinical trials. CR Clinical is also dedicated to educating individuals and providing job opportunities in clinical research.

Please visit www.crclinical.com to learn about CR Clinical and what we offer!

www.ingramcontent.com/pod-product-compliance
Lightning Source LLC
Chambersburg PA
CBHW072019230526
45479CB00008B/297